The Motion Sickness Relief Handbook

Includes 20 Wacky (and Not Such Wacky) Ways to Prevent or Overcome Motion Sickness

Indie Penn

ISBN: 9781707286874

DEDICATION

This book is dedicated to myself, a person who has battled motion sickness since birth.

CONTENTS

IMPORTANT NOTE

The material presented here is for informational purposes only.   The tips, tricks, ideas and techniques in this book are not intended to be a substitute for consultation and treatment by a qualified healthcare professional. I make no guarantee that the information in this book will prevent or relieve any form of motion sickness. The content presented here is based mainly on my own experience with travel nausea.   It is not necessarily scientifically or medically proven to be accurate or effective. Do not implement these strategies unless approved by a qualified health care professional.

INTRODUCTION

You will notice that I keep on referring to car sickness throughout this work, and don't focus so much on the other modes of travel that bring on motion sickness, like airplanes, cruise ships, trains and amusement rides. Despite the fact that I use cars and vehicles as the main subject of this work, most of the principles and techniques I discuss here can be adapted to any form of travel and most motion rides. If you cannot see how a particular idea can be utilized in a particular motion ride then you can safely assume that the particular idea is only relevant to car travel.

If all the theories I discuss in chapters one or two bore you to death, feel free to skip it all and go straight to the beef in chapter three.

CHAPTER 1
CAUSE OF MOTION SICKNESS

What causes motion sickness?

It is my opinion that our bodies like be in a position of "comfort" at all times. Body's favorite position? Comfort. Any time that that comfort is threatened, physically or emotionally, our bodies will react in one way or another.

Many of our bodies, definitely my body, will produce physical symptoms any time it feels its comfortable position to be threatened.

Since most of us are not born in moving vehicles-thank God!-and don't spend much of our early days in them, when we do get into a car our bodies feel uncomfortable and react by getting us to become nauseous or dizzy.

Think about it. All day long, since the day you were born, you were basically creating your own movement. You moved your arms and legs, you flipped onto your stomach and back, you walked, you ran…you get the idea.

And even when you had movement created for you, when you were rocked in your crib or in your parent's arms, when you were pushed on a swing, when you were carried by the adults around you, you were still pretty much in control of your field of vision. You basically saw the same scene, the same objects as you were rocked in your crib or pushed on the swing. When you were carried around by a parent, and even when you were wheeled around in your stroller, the scene in front of you did keep on changing, but none of this compares to the *type* of movement and *type* of visual exposure you are subjected to when you ride in a vehicle.

Now suddenly, one day, you are strapped into a car. You get moved around for a long time in a funny way. Depending on the vehicle, you're either being bumped around, vibrated around or just slid around in a weird up and down way. And as you try to process these new sensations, you are seeing scores of objects whiz by you per minute. Here's a red sports car, here's a black jeep, here's a blue motorcycle, here's a little house and another house and a tree and another tree and another tree and a deer, and a tire... Your body is confused and uncomfortable with this out-of-comfort-zone experience.

In the past, when you experienced movement, the scenery around you did not change much. If it did, it changed at a slow pace and your body was able to adjust to these changes gradually. Slowly it would make itself comfortable. But now your body is *experiencing* a completely different sort of motion. At the same time, it's *hearing* the hum of the motor and *seeing* so many different objects fly by at such a fast pace. There's so much sensory feedback that your body needs to process simultaneously. Your body is feeling totally messed up. Disorientation sets in. Your body's kind of panicking. Its likely response? Nausea or/and dizziness.

As a child of about ten years old I decided I wanted to start reading books in bed. My mother never introduced me to that idea so I must've picked it up from friends or books! Whatever the cause, I started this new routine enthusiastically, but how odd it was, that on night number one of this new routine, I felt myself sweating and was overcome with nausea. I remember putting away the book, but the nausea lingered. I was feeling horrible. At some point or other I fell asleep.

Determined as ever, I was right back to reading in bed on night number two. Again, the same thing happened. I became sweaty and nauseous. I tried reading in bed for another couple of days, then promptly gave up my newfound habit. And I was back to sleeping like a log!

Sometime in my teenage years, I decided to try again to read myself to sleep. Same thing happened. After reading a page or two, I was beginning to feel the nausea set in. But this time I wasn't a kid. As a thoughtful teenager I thought into this strange phenomena, and I thought some more, until I came up with the following theory.

When I put myself into bed to sleep, my body goes into relaxation mode. As part of the relaxation mode I ease up on my logical thinking. I let my mind wander and unleash my imagination. This is what I've exposed myself to for a number of years of my life.

Then suddenly, one nice moonlit night, I decide to take up reading in bed. Here my body is slowly releasing all pent up tension, dimming the logic and here I am, at the very same time, trying to stimulate the logical part in my brain. This disorients my body and as a result, guess what? You can guess, right? I'm nauseous!

Interestingly, other members of my family have had similar experiences. My brother, Josh, used to vomit on occasion right before he went to sleep. It wasn't a virus or anything, and he always felt perfectly fine the next day.

At first it seemed completely randomized, but then over time my mother noticed an interesting pattern. Any time Jack was overtired, usually due to him missing his regular bedtime, he would become nauseous and vomit.

The reason according to my theory? Josh's body is crying for sleep. It's winding down. But as it's winding down, Josh is obstinately trying to wind it up. The result? Physical reaction; in his case it was nausea.

I must say that I continue to see this happening, now with some of my own children. If they are overhyped just before their bedtime or if they miss their bedtime by more than one hour, they frequently come out of bed tearfully complaining that they are nauseous.

Telling them to return to bed would be counterintuitive. It would be like sending a person suffering from road sickness right back into a car. Instead I tell them to forget about going to sleep. I give them some ice cubes to suck on and tell them to go do an activity they like, like reading, coloring or writing.

Now the body is no longer in conflict. It's no longer getting mixed messages of "wind down when you are all wound up". Instead we expose the body to a routine daytime activity. This lets the body wind down gradually, in a way it is familiar with. The body is then returned to its comfort level and so are my kids. After a while they'll just feel better and return to their beds.

Why do only some people get motion sickness?

You might be thinking, *very nice theory and all but why doesn't everybody get motion sickness? Why is riding in a vehicle torturous for some and completely fun for others?*

I'm going to challenge you to another question in order to answer your question.

Why do only some children develop allergies to certain things?

Why are some children unable to breathe when exposed to peanuts while others walk around blissfully with their peanut butter sandwiches?

Due to our different genetic makeups, each of our bodies perceive different things as a threat to its comfort based on the particular processing system God endowed it with. We each have a completely unique processing system, pretty much unique as our fingerprint.

And you know what happens when your stomach doesn't process a particular food well. You get to feel quite uncomfortable for a while, whether in the form of heartburn, gas or stomach ache.

Your body works the same way. If your body finds it difficult to adapt to a particular new sensation, experience or food well, then it goes into a discomfort zone. Once in discomfort, the body may react physically by inducing nausea, dizziness, hives, rashes, coughs, headaches, backaches, toothaches, TMJ, muscular pain or other uncomfortable, painful and sometimes even dangerous conditions.

When my body is introduced to a new food, it generally processes the food perfectly well. I hardly land up with an allergic reaction to the food I ate. However, changes in position are not processed well by my body at all. For me, looking downward from a high elevation induces vertigo, riding any merry go round style amusement park ride makes me dizzy and of course riding in a car, even for only ten minutes or so, can bring on horrible nausea.

What about the people you know who never have any physical reaction to anything?

I would say that this group of people has one of two things going for them. Either they have fantastic, state of the art processing systems (that's not to say that their lives are more perfect or more stress free than yours; it just means that they tend to suffer less from physical aches and pains.) or they are never exposed to the things that would not be processed well by their bodies. In other words, their processing system is a very good fit for the sensations, experiences or foods that they happen to be exposed to quite regularly.

It's possible that one of those perfect people you know would become dizzy at certain elevations. However, since he is not a mountain climber he may never be exposed to that elevation in his lifetime.

My baby has traveled in a car since birth. Why is she suddenly vomiting at one year old?

You might be from the thousands of people who are in and out of cars all day. In this case your baby has been exposed to traveling in a vehicle since birth. Why then does your baby suddenly vomit in the car at one years old?

So first I have to tell you that I believe that a child who is in and out of a car constantly since birth is less likely to develop motion sickness. I have not seen any studies **stating that this is indeed the case; it's just my guess based on how we humans operate**.

What about the babies who do begin vomiting at age one or two?

Well, do you know that until about three to four months old a baby can only see up to one foot, yep that's only twelve inches, ahead? And it's only in the fifth month that a baby begins to see the world as a three dimensional place. In fact, according to the American Optometric Association it can take until the age of two for a child's depth perception (that means a three dimensional view of the world) to be completely developed.

So it is no wonder that a child's brain suddenly becomes overwhelmed by travel at age one or two. While previously the baby might have not seen anything out the window, and might have focused completely on the handle of his car seat for the duration of his ride, at two years of age the entire traveling experience takes on a completely new dimension. He now perceives car travel in a similar way to adults.

CHAPTER 2
TREATING MOTION SICKNESS

Now that we understand the cause of motion sickness, we can go ahead and attempt to treat it.

There are three different ways we can treat motion sickness.

1. TREATING THE SYMPTOM

In this treatment we work on eliminating the nausea and/or dizziness that our bodies produce in response to its discomfort. It's kind of like treating a bacterial infection with antibiotics. We are healing the infection but not necessarily the cause of the infection. This treatment is similar also to the way we treat allergies.

When a person has an allergy that is not life threatening, generally the first course of treatment is to take Benadryl. Benadryl is an antihistamine, which means it blocks the effect that histamine has on the body. Histamine is the actual horrible "thingy" that a body produces when it feels its comfort threatened. This thingy causes all those uncomfortable and/or dangerous allergy associated conditions.

So you see, Benadryl blocks the effect that allergies have on a person but it is helpless in getting the body not to see a particular food or particle as an allergy, as an enemy, in the first place.

Nausea really is a form of an allergic reaction. Our body doesn't like something and as a result, it will produce the physical symptom of nausea and/or dizziness.

Dramimine, an over the counter medication that many people take before traveling so they don't get motion sickness, works in a similar way to Benadryl. It blocks the effect that histamine has on the body. It doesn't let the histamine complete its task of getting you nauseous or dizzy.

So preventing the histamine (and other substances that our bodies release to make us feel sick) from negatively effecting us is one way in which we can free ourselves from suffering from motion sickness.

2. ELIMINATING THE CAUSE (VIA EXPOSURE)

Wouldn't it be amazing if we could stop motion sickness from starting in the first place? Well we could. And the way to do that is through training our bodies that car travel is not a threat. We want to let our bodies know that traveling in a vehicle is a wonderful, relaxing and comfortable experience.

So how do we do that? Our bodies are extremely sensitive, extremely stubborn and oh so smart. But the fact is that we own our own brains and with wisdom we can convince our bodies that traveling really is a wonderful experience.

The most effective way to train our bodies to a new comfort is to force the body to try this new comfort for a very long time.

Remember the time you were introduced to this weird new dish? You tasted it and your senses were overwhelmed by the strong, weird taste. I bet you never tried it again, certainly not for a long time. However, if you would have continued to try that dish again and again, you may have come to love it or, at the least, to tolerate it soon enough.

Actually most alcoholics do not like their first drink much, but they try it again and again until they become addicted.

This is kind of the way exposure therapy works. In exposure therapy, one of the most popular and successful mental health therapy techniques, a person is introduced to the trigger of his phobia or fear again and again until he becomes desensitized, and his trigger fails to be a trigger of fear any longer.

Let's take somebody who is afraid of dogs. A psychologist will recommend that he go to a park during off-leash hours and take a nice walk while scores of dogs run around loosely. At first he'll have the fright of his life but after doing it consistently, time and time again, he will lose his fear of dogs.

Exposure therapy is available in two different tracks. Track one is called gradual exposure therapy. Yep, you guessed correctly. In this track the person is gradually exposed to the trigger of his phobia. In the case of the person who is afraid of dogs, he will first practice passing leashed dogs again and again. Then he might expose himself to an unleashed dog, which is under the supervision of its owner and eventually he would expose himself to a full field of unleashed dogs.

The second track a person may choose to follow for his exposure therapy is called flooding. Flooding is simply the opposite of gradual exposure therapy. In this method the person floods all his senses with his fear. He walks straight into a field full of unleashed dogs and despite his absolute terror he does not leave the park for a long while. He does this again, evening after evening. And in a very short time his fear of dogs just dissipates.

If car travel plays a big role in your life, you might just want to try exposure therapy. To be totally honest, I've never personally tried exposure therapy for motion sickness because traveling simply doesn't play such a large role in my life. There are quite a number of phobias that I have that I know I can heal via exposure therapy. However, since I don't frequent those triggers often enough, I just won't bother.

Loose dogs is one such a phobia that I possess. How often do I frequent a loose dog? Not often at all; so why bother to address that fear. I won't tell you about the time I nearly passed out when I tried running away from a loose dog. (By the way, you can hardly ever outrun a dog so don't even try!)

However, if you feel like your quality of life is significantly affected by your motion sickness, I do encourage you to experiment with exposure therapy. I cannot imagine that it will not work for at least most bad travelers.

Let's go back to our allergy comparison.

Just a short while back, the standardized treatment for food and air allergies was avoidance. If you were allergic to nuts, you just stayed away from them. If you were allergic to seasonal allergies, you just tried to stay indoors when pollen counts are high.

In recent years treatment of allergies has changed to gradual exposure therapy. Today you can buy nut patches to gradually introduce nuts to a child who is allergic to them. Gradual exposure therapy is used for allergies as opposed to flooding because flooding might bring a child to a life threatening physical condition. (**Caution**: nut patches or any form of exposure may be life threatening to a child and/or person who is severely allergic to a particular allergen. In these cases no form of exposure should be introduced or experimented with unless it is under the care of a qualified health care professional.)

If you are allergic to things in the air, like pollen, dust or mold, you might consider taking allergy shots. These injections expose you to a tiny bit of your allergen and with time you are supposed to be able to tolerate the air around you better.

It's interesting that when I discussed these allergy shots with my mother, she told me she thought it was a perfectly stupid thing to take. She told me that my father suffered from seasonal allergies for years and then it was gone. Actually many people have had that experience. They just kind of outgrew their seasonal allergies. What does it mean? It just means that they were subjected to natural exposure therapy. Over years of being exposed to seasonal allergies, their bodies finally became comfortable with them and stopped triggering histamine when they were exposed to them.

Let's get back to discussing motion sickness now.

If it means a lot to you to stop getting motion sickness, if you're on the road or sea often, if your income or hobby is dependent on travel, you might want to subject yourself to flooding.

Here's how.

Move into a car (or a truck, boat, airplane, train) for a month. Don't get out when you start getting sick because that defeats the purpose of the exposure therapy. Stay in there through all your nausea, vomiting and dizziness. Stay in there until you stop having any symptoms at all. And then you should be healed.

Now once healed, if you don't step into a car for a long while again, your motion sickness might restart because your body won't recognize car travel anymore. So, to maintain your gains, make sure to get into a vehicle very often and eventually, my guess is, you will be healed for years.

I would say that exposure therapy is the most difficult way to get out of motion sickness, but it is also the most effective. You can actually heal yourself completely by forcing your body to become comfortable with car travel.

I am certain that if we would be born in cars and live in cars, instead of houses, when we would leave our car once in a while, many of us would experience some uncomfortable physical symptoms. So if you spend a good deal of life on the road, you can simulate a born-in-a-car, live-in-a-car lifestyle to make your body comfortable with the idea of riding in a car, and you might just get stationary sickness when you decide to get out!

NOTE: Before implementing the flooding technique for motion sickness make sure to read Trick 20 in Chapter three of this work. In Trick 20 I provide more detail about how to apply the flooding technique so that it has the desired effect.

3. ELIMINATING THE CAUSE (VIA DECEPTION)

While the results of exposure therapy should be fantastic, it is a very intense treatment to go through. If you're a chicken like me and don't want to go through all of that, you might want to make your body comfortable with riding in a car via deception and distraction.

What we want to do is prevent our bodies from becoming overwhelmed by everything that goes on when riding a car. If our senses won't become overwhelmed then our bodies are likely to stay in their comfort zones and there would be no good reason for them to make us feel nauseous or dizzy.

So how do we do that?

Over the years I've come up with tips and tricks to get my body to focus so intensely on a single one of my senses that it becomes completely distracted from my traveling and continues to feel safe and comfortable even during travel. For example, when riding a bus I will stand in the aisle without holding on to any seats or rails. This forces my body to focus all its energies and thoughts on maintaining my balance. It's crazy and not very comfortable but it does keep the travel nausea at bay. It's not my favorite technique at all and there are way better ways to keep your body in its comfort zone. I'll be sharing more of these crazy tricks with you soon. You'll be glad to know that many of them are quite simple and comfortable to travel with.

Now none of these tricks will heal you from motion sickness, you're not going to get your body to adapt and become truly comfortable with vehicle travel, but you will be able to travel comfortably one trip at a time, as long as your body continues to fall for your distractions.

When these tricks don't work, it means that your body is not engaged enough for long enough by the trick you tried. Then it is free to refocuses its attention on the car movement. In this case, you need to come up with other tricks that are more engaging and riveting, to grab your body's focus away from car travel.

It's interesting to note that motion sickness is much less common in the driver's seat. You are less likely to become nauseous if you are the driver of the vehicle than if you are the passenger. This is because as a driver you are controlling the car and are fully immersed in the movement. So your body is not a victim to confusion. It is fully occupied in planning and creating the movement. That's so much less disorienting for your body and a less disoriented body, means a more comfortable body which means a more comfortable you!

CHAPTER 3
20 TIPS AND TRICKS

In this chapter I am going to introduce you to 20 tips and tricks that can help you avoid or overcome travel nausea. Every trick I share here either treats the symptoms of motion sickness or eliminates the cause of motion sickness via deception, distraction or adaption. Tighten your seatbelts and hang on tight as we explore both the mainstream and the wacky ways to find relief from travel sickness.

1. DRAMIMINE

Dramimine used to be the brand name for the over the counter medication Dymenhydrinate only. Today however the Dramimine brand produces 3 main products for nausea and each of those contain a different main ingredient.

a. Dramimine Original
This Dramimine formula contains Dymenhydrinate as its main drug.

b. Dramimine Less Drowsy
Last I've checked this Dramimine contained the drug Meclizine as its main drug.

c. Dramimine Non Drowsy
Whoa! Dramimine has joined the world of natural medicine. Non Drowsy Dramimine contains natural ginger as its main ingredient, an herb believed to prevent and relieve nausea.

Dramimine works as an antihistamine. That means it blocks the histamine that your body produces as a result of its discomfort, and does not allow that histamine to have a negative effect on you. Dramimine is generally taken about a half hour before traveling and lasts for about 6-8 hours. There's also an All Day formula that lasts for about 24 hours. Note: Chewable Dramimine is available for children.

For my husband, myself and our children, Dramimine usually works well in preventing nausea. However, I do sometimes become slightly dizzy, even when I'm on Dramimine. I also sometimes get delayed motion sickness, where I will become slightly queasy or nauseous once I'm finished traveling and I'm off the medicine. I believe that both of these symptoms, slight dizziness during travel and a delayed physical reaction to travel, come because my body tries to react to its discomfort in ways that are possible for it to react.

Remember we said that Dramimine only blocks the effect histamine has on the body but it doesn't prevent the body from reacting in the first place? My belief is that since my body cannot possibly get me to become nauseous as a result of its discomfort, due to the Dramimine effect, it pulls a different trigger and gets me to react with slight dizziness. Or it brings on the reaction to its discomfort later, once I am already off the medicine and can no longer fight the histamine effect.

Who cares though? I'd rather feel a bit dizzy and unsteady than feel nauseous anytime! And feeling slightly queasy or woozy in bed after a long trip is not really a big deal. I fall asleep fast enough and sleep off any residual motion sickness.

Remember I mentioned that the Original Dramimine and the Less Drowsy Dramimine contain completely different main drugs?

I didn't monitor the nausea relieving results of the Less Drowsy version for long enough, but I did notice that the few times Dramimine didn't have a perfect effect on us was when we took the Less Drowsy version. However, I can't be certain that the original formula did work one hundred percent of the time so none of this is conclusive. I recently began tracking the results of both the Original and the Less Drowsy formula. Once I have tracked it for long enough I will include an update here, in an updated version of this book. What was your experience with the different Dramimine formulas available on the market? I'd love to hear! My email address is: indiepenn@gmail.com.

The first time I was serious about taking Dramimine was when I was a senior in high school. For our senior trip we were going to spend a day at Niagara Falls. Don't ask me who on the staff came up with this ridiculous idea but we were going to travel throughout the night, spend the day at the falls, and return to New York at night. That means about ten hours of travel, two nights in a row. As a terrible traveler, I let my classmates know that I was not joining them. Well, they wouldn't accept it at all. Missing the senior annual trip was a no-no and nobody could understand why I would choose to miss a major trip for such a dumb reason. Only really bad travelers can relate to that mindset. So after a tremendous amount of pressure that came from both my classmates and some of my teachers! I agreed to join. And then promptly went about looking for a solution to my motion sickness.

Here and there I tried the chewable Dramimine as I was never really able to swallow pills. I found the taste to be horrible and it actually triggered a nausea reaction before I even got into a vehicle. This time I was determined to get the Dramimine down my system the right way. My desperation actually taught me how to swallow pills, not in the conventional way but in a way that it worked just as well. I don't want to get you nauseous so I won't elaborate on the details of my pill swallowing affair. I'll just say it went something like this: Getting the pill into the center of mashed up pretzels (not saying how they got mashed up), then swallowing the pretzel mush in the regular conventional way you'd swallow pretzels.

The trip was a wild success for me. I took the pills religiously every six hours, as per package instructions, and did not get nauseous!

Now that doesn't sound like much of a story, definitely not one that is fit to be printed. Right?

Well, here's the punch.

On the second night of our trip we were all totally exhausted. We hadn't had any shuteye at all the night before as we partied away on the bus. We had spent the entire day running from one attraction to the next. By the time night fell we were spent.

I took my last dose of Dramimine and fell into a deep sleep. At some point I awoke from my sleep, feeling horribly nauseous. I peeked at my watch and couldn't believe it. It was just the time for my next dosage. I grabbed another pill out of somewhere and fell asleep again. By the time we hit home, I woke up feeling perfectly fine. Well hey, I was still under Dramimine's effect. It wasn't the time yet for my next dose!

This story enlightened me to just how real motion sickness is. Even in my sleep it took effect!

You might ask how that is even possible. We blamed some of motion sickness on vision and the truth is that vision and focus do play a big role in motion sickness. Nearly everybody who suffers from motion sickness will admit that reading while riding is a sure way to get the nausea to come fast and strong. So what was it?

Remember I told you about my brother Josh who vomited just before he went to bed when he was past his bedtime?

Well that may very well be the cause for motion sickness during our sleep. Here our body is trying to sleep. It's in a place of almost complete relaxation, but the atmosphere is completely off. It's sensing the coach bus smell (in my case), it's hearing this weird humming sound, it's feeling itself being bumped about in all sorts of different ways. It is no wonder at all that the sleeping passenger develops nausea!

After this trip I was sold on Dramimine. I took it any time I traveled long distances and finally I was able to enjoy my car rides and the scenery around me as I traveled!

Sometimes Dramimine doesn't work perfectly and I do develop a hint of nausea. As I mentioned earlier, I believe that the Original formula is more effective than the Less Drowsy. Though the Dramimine brand produces both formulas each formula is a completely different drug so it is logical to assume that one drug works better than the other, or that certain people respond better to certain drugs.

Another aspect to consider is that I've never yet taken more than one Dramimine pill at a time, even though the package recommends taking one to two pills every four to six hours. **Note:** By the time you read this book Dramimine may have already changed their dosage recommendations so always read the medicine packaging before determining your exact dosage.

The downside of Dramimine, other than the fact that it is a medicine, is that many users complain about the super drowsy effect it has on them. Personally, I'll take extreme drowsiness, even sleep, over nausea but everybody's different. However I must say that the Original formula does not result in a very intense drowsiness for me. I feel a bit drowsy and lethargic but I function way better when I'm drowsy than when I feel nauseous.

A personal downside of the children's chewable Dramimine is that my children absolutely hate the taste of it. Getting them to take it is no simple feat. Usually they end up half chewing it and half spitting it out and then try to prove to me that the Dramimine didn't work! So I do hope your kids' taste buds are more receptive to the Dramimine pill. If so, then the downside of the chewable Dramimine remains totally personal to me!

As in all drugs, always talk to your qualified health professional before trying it and follow the packaging instructions!

You notice I didn't talk much about the Non Drowsy formula. Over the years I've read a lot about the effectiveness of ginger as a nausea relief solution but was never really convinced that it worked. So I just never tried it. That's the truth. I never tried the Non Drowsy formula.

It's interesting to compare the reviews on Amazon.com of the Original and Less Drowsy Dramimine (which Amazon currently has under one listing) and the ginger filled Non Drowsy Dramimine.

Only 5 percent of all reviewers for the Original/Less Drowsy formula gave it a negative one star review, while a whopping 15 percent reviewers gave the ginger Dramimine a negative one star review!

If you actually read through the one star reviews on the Original/Less drowsy formula you will see that most reviewers are only complaining that they received poor quality pills or knockoffs. The few reviews that claim that the Dramimine didn't work at all are reviews left about the Less Drowsy or chewable version of Dramimine.

Most of the one star reviews on the ginger version though complain about the pill not working at all!

My feeling is that ginger is not anywhere as effective as the Original and Less Drowsy version of Dramimine.

I believe that many people find relief from chewing or sucking ginger flavored products or drinking ginger flavored tea. It's possible that ginger might work better on the taste buds than in the bloodstream.

If you are a naturalist or you have a specific reason you cannot take the Original or Less Drowsy Dramimine then you might just want to give the ginger version a shot. Or you might prepare yourself a travel bag of ginger flavored products. Hey, you never know!

2. SCOPOLAMINE PATCHES

Scopolamine patches, sold under the brand name Transderm Scop, are meant to be placed behind the ears. Slowly, over 3 days, it releases a medication into the body that blocks the effect that nausea inducing substances (that your body creates as a result of feeling displaced) have on the central nervous system.

While it is in a different class of drugs than Dramimine, it works in a similar way, by blocking nausea inducing substances from having an ill effect on you.

The downside of these patches is that it is not an over the counter medicine. You need to get a prescription from a doctor for it.

It is great however for long trips and cruises because once stuck onto your skin it does not need to be touched for the next three days. It's waterproof as well.

I have never tried it personally but it seems that many people have experienced great relief when using these patches.

3. SING YOUR HEART OUT

For some reason singing my heart out just relaxes my body and takes it into a super comfort zone. And, mind you, I am most unmusical and partially tone deaf, I think. I don't play music nor do I listen to music much. Despite it all, any time I spend my trip singing soulful songs that I like I just don't get nauseous.

But here's the thing. You need to sing with enthusiasm, with all your heart. Make believe you are directing a concert. Maybe get yourself a baton to dramatize the singing. Put your whole self into it. If you're going to just *do* the singing, then it's just not going to work.

I discovered this trick by accident. I began noticing that any time I traveled with my friends and we sang I just wouldn't get nauseous. If the singing stopped midway, then a short while later the nausea would set in. If I wouldn't be totally ashamed I would have just continued to sing solo for the rest of the ride. But the shame…I just couldn't do it.

Now, when I travel with my family I turn on a nice CD and I lead a beautiful traveling choir. My kids told me that indeed singing prevents them from getting nauseous.

So why not try it out. It's pretty much free (unless you buy a baton) and completely natural.

4. LEAVE THE WINDOWS OPEN

If you can, get the car to drive fast (within the speed limit, of course!), open all the windows, shut off the heat or air conditioning and let yourself feel the natural air swirling all around you.

This should send a signal to your body that you are not in some indoor place where everything is stationary. You're out somewhere in the not so predictable world, where sensations and experiences vary. When your body gets that idea it might not panic that you're being jolted around.

Make sure you receive the fullest benefit of the open window as possible. Get a seat where the window opens completely, if you can.

5. SNIFF ORANGE JUICE

Okay, this is a weird one, I admit. I came up with this out of desperation. I live in New York and use the subway a lot to get into the city. I often travel with a large stroller and need to use the subway elevators. The elevators though smell bad, really bad. They are constantly cleaned but somehow they often smell so bad that if I'd be there any longer than how long it takes to ride an elevator, I'd vomit. For sure.

Finally, I came up with a solution. On one of my trips in to the city, I brought along a small orange juice drink and as soon as I entered the elevator I almost dunked my nose into the juice. I smelled and smelled the lovely scent of fresh orange juice. It was blissful.

Since that first wonderful orange juice experience, I make sure to take along beverages that I like with strong, pleasant smells whenever I ride the city's elevators.

This worked so well for elevators, I decided to try it in travel as well. When I enter cars or buses, especially coach buses that have a very strong nausea inducing smell (for me, at least), I sniff my precious orange juice. If the smell is strong enough, you can forget somewhat that you are in a vehicle.

The downside of this is that it's not really all that exciting to keep on sniffing for hours. After a while, even if you're still holding the orange juice bottle to your nose or dunking your nose into the orange juice you really forget to sniff and start focusing on other things. So this really is a good trick for short rides. For longer rides I do not recommend it.

For me the smell and taste of orange juice is very refreshing, but everybody's got their own preferences. You don't need to use orange juice. Try lemonade, try a container of coffee beans, take along a couple of perfume bottles, whatever it is that appeals to your sense of smell. Just remember it needs to be a really fresh and invigorating smell for you, not just some okay, pleasant smell.

My kids absolutely love this idea and it keeps them distracted for quite some time when in the car. You might want to bring along a "scent bag" with all sorts of different smells and keep on passing them around. We once owned a Bing Bong plush doll from Disney with a heavenly cotton candy scent. That scent for us was lovely and so refreshing, and the scent held on for years. I haven't seen that doll around for a while but it might still carry that lovely scent. If you can get each of your kids such a plush for travel it could very well act as a real body relaxant and you might just avoid having to deal with nauseous and vomiting kids.

6. TAKE OVER CONTROL

If you've got your driver's license and are comfortable at the wheel, choose to be the driver. Most drivers don't suffer from motion sickness.

What if you don't drive or cannot possibly be the driver?

Then be in control of the entertainment! Make it your business to take care of all technicalities from food and drink distribution to fun and road spirit. You might want to think of yourself as the steward.

This will keep your mind so preoccupied with activities it is familiar with that it might not mind the riding part at all.

The downside of this is that it is only possible to implement when you are with a group of people *and* you're on a bus, train or airplane. If you're squashed into a car there's really not much you can do, and doing just a little bit of entertaining will not get you anywhere.

But anytime you're on a bus, promote yourself to supervisor. Even if you're with strangers you can walk around to chat with people and offer them drinks, refreshments and entertainment. Make sure to include the driver as well or he'll order you off the bus…

7. STAND ALL THE TIME

My son travels by coach bus often and refuses to take Dramimine. Instead he stands in the aisle for the entire duration of his trip (about one and a half hours!), and he finds that that most often keeps him from getting nauseous.

It's pretty logical that standing and working on maintaining your balance as you ride a vehicle will keep you from developing motion sickness. It should make perfect logical sense to your body. You're focused on maintaining your balance because it's being offset by the traveling bus. That's much less disorienting than sitting and relaxing and having your body experience all sorts of movements and sights that really match better with a standing and moving experience.

Again this is something you can only implement on a bus though.

8. FACE FORWARD ONLY

Sitting backwards is the absolute worst position for a traveler who is prone to motion sickness. I remember the days of the station wagon, when all of us kids would be settled onto those side facing benches in the back of the car. I don't think I ever did NOT get nauseous.

Sitting backward is really horrible for our poor bodies that are already overwhelmed by so many different signals at once!

So you are sitting facing forward. Now make sure you don't glance out of any side windows. Make sure you don't read or text or do any sort of technical activity. Just keep your eyes on the horizon. The entire time.

Looking out the front window is the absolute best way to treat our sensitive bodies. This is almost similar to controlling the wheel of the car. Our bodies have a chance to anticipate which objects will be passing us before they do. It is most similar to non-car travel living.

If you are traveling by airplane, make sure you keep the window shutters closed. Looking out of those side windows is the surest way to confuse your body and get you sick. There's no way to convince your body that it is in a completely comfortable spot when you're up there in the clouds so the best thing you can do is try to convince your body that it is not moving at all, that you are just in a room with stale air.

If you don't have a seat right near the airplane window, you cannot really control the window shades. That's why I like aisle seats. That enables me not to notice the open shutters. I try to focus on the small area around me. I'll even read on an airplane because I don't really feel the movement at all, once the plane is in cruising phase. Only turbulence and open window shutters will get me to become nauseous on an airplane.

9. MIST BOTTLES

Get a couple of mist spray bottles. Keep them cold. Once on the road, when you begin feeling a bit queasy, spray your face with ice cold mist. It's a heavenly sensation that can pull your body back to a place of comfort.

If you've got a couple of people with you, you can have fun spraying each other up. There'll be so much fun and laughter, that if you can maintain this for the duration for your trip I think every single rider will avoid motion sickness.

10. INSTANT COLD PACKS

This is similar to the mist bottle technique, only more sensational and less fun. When you begin feeling just a bit queasy, activate a few instant ice packs and press it at your temples, forehead and/or neck. (Don't hold it on any area for too long or it could be dangerous to your health. Follow packaging instructions.)

This will shock your system out of its discomfort and disorientation and send a message of comfort and rejuvenation to your system. It might just trick your system into forgetting about its discomfort altogether.

11. SUPER HOT TEA

Another way to shock your system out of its discomfort and disorientation is to treat yourself to a piping hot coffee or tea. There's just something very comforting and shocking and rejuvenating in a hot drink.

Electric car kettles are extremely popular today and are quite inexpensive to buy. This kettle will allow you to prepare hot drinks inside your car at your whim, so you don't need to stop anywhere and spend money.

Take Caution! Make sure the drinks are not too hot when passed around in the car. If you are traveling with children this might not be the best technique to try.

12. LET YOURSELF GET CHILLY

This really is only applicable when you travel in cold weather. Instead of turning up the heat, which for me is always a motion sickness trigger, let your vehicle stay cold. Open the windows to let the cold air in. The colder it is, the more energy your body will need to dispense to keep you warm and it will be completely preoccupied with this task. You are not likely to get nauseous.

If the cold is really uncomfortable for you, you might try this for short periods of time, as you feel yourself getting nauseous. Then, when you feel better, you can close the windows and turn on the heat.

Take Caution! Extreme cold can cause dangerous health conditions and even death. Make sure that the weather is not too cold to put you or anybody who is traveling with you at risk.

I have found this technique to work incredibly well for me. How I love the shivers when I travel. It means no nausea!

The downside of this is that your travel companions might not appreciate this at all. For somebody who is a great traveler, there's nothing like a warm, toasty car in the dead of the winter.

13. PRESSING YOUR TEMPLES

As you feel yourself getting dizzy or nauseous, use your finger to gently press your temples. For some reason that sensation can move your body back into comfort zone.

If you are traveling with family or friends you might all grab a partner and do the temple pressing for each other. That makes for a fun, nausea relieving team activity.

I have found that this works only some of the time. But try it, you've got nothing to lose.

14. CARBONATED DRINKS

If you're slightly nauseous, grab a highly carbonated drink that you like. Take a couple of gulps and burp as strong and fast as you can. Burping is a substitute for vomiting and you might just convince your body that it accomplished its task and has gotten you to vomit. Then you'll feel better.

The downside to this is that the drinks I buy are never as carbonated as I like. I find that the small soda cans are best – the plastic bottles just never are as fizzy – but I wish they'd give me more burping material.

Another issue is that once you open the can and take a couple of gulps, you cannot close it and all the fizz goes out. So for each set of burps, you're going to need a new soda can, which is not all that bad and definitely worth the money considering that it can prevent you from vomiting.

Happy Burping!

15. THICK SALTY PRETZELS

Ever since we were little kids, whenever we complained of car sickness my mother would distribute thick salty pretzels. There's something very soothing about them. I would guess that the salt on our taste buds shock our poor, confused bodies back into a place of comfort.

You know how pacifiers just get an agitated baby to relax? I like to think of these thick salty pretzels as pacifiers for those suffering from motion sickness.

16. FREQUENT STOPS

Keep on stopping and getting out of your car for fresh air. It will prolong your trip but keep you comfortable the entire time.

When you do this, you just won't be in the car for long enough to have the nausea set in. By the time your body starts producing all that horrible stuff that make you sick, you'll be out of the car, and your body will hopefully withdraw its reaction.

This can be turned into something fun, if you choose to stop at cool places. If you're traveling with children, you might stop off at parks and/or different entertainment centers. If you're traveling with adults you might stop off at some malls or shopping centers. And who doesn't love food? Everybody will love a stop at a restaurant!

17. GRAB A FRONT SEAT

Make it your business to get a seat that is as close as possible to the front of the vehicle. The closer you are to the front windows, the less disoriented your body is likely to become. The best seat of course is the front passenger seat, right beside the driver.

18. GET A MASSAGE

Since our bodies get confused by the sensory feedback they receive from traveling it would be wonderful if we can have them focus on *different* sensory feedback instead.

Getting a full body massage over and over again as you travel will force your body to focus on more comfortable and recognizable sensations. You would be forcing your body to choose between focusing on the primary sensory feedback it's getting - the massage, or the secondary sensory input it's getting - the car movement. I suggest that during the massage you close your eyes and get into a comfortable position so you don't confuse your body with your field of vision —fast moving and fast changing scenery — as it attempts to adjust to the wonderful massage it is getting.

There are all kind of cool handheld massage machines on the market. Best is if you can have a traveling companion give you the massage. If that's not practical you can get machines that you can work on your own, like foot massagers, neck and shoulder massagers, and you can even get a wearable cape that massages you with vibrations!

19. CHOOSE THE RIGHT VEHICLE

For some reason different bodies respond differently to different motions, even to subtle differences.

Personally all of us, my children and I, ride horribly on coach buses. It is absolutely the worst mode of travel for us. We all agree that those yellow school buses are way friendlier to our delicate bodies than these fancy coach buses.

I also find that I will get nauseous faster in a car with a low roof than I will in a vehicle that is more elevated, like a minivan or just any sleek, slightly elevated car. I did however hear people complain that SUV's get them very nauseous. I don't have much personal experience with those.

It is possible that a body that has ridden more often in a nice comfortable car might get overwhelmed on the occasions that it rides in a nice comfortable SUV. That's because it has already adapted somewhat to the car motion but not to the SUV motion. I ride in different minivans a lot so it could be that my body has adapted somewhat to minivans but goes into complete discomfort when forced into a low roofed car!

We all love trains! I don't get nauseous in them (so long as I don't read or sit facing the back of the train) and none of my children get nauseous in them either. It is fairly unusual to get nauseous on most trains as the movement and general experience is very different from the unpredictable movement present in a vehicle on the road.

We also love the big ferry boat in New York City that we sometime take a short ride with. We don't generally get sick on it but our rides are always very short. It is possible that if we'd travel deep out into the open sea, we'd suffer extreme seasickness. Many passengers who travel on cruises tend to get very seasick.

Vehicles that smell of car fresheners or motors instantly get me nauseous. I believe that is because my body associates these smells with travel and motion sickness so upon exposure to that smell it falls right into discomfort zone. Many travelers claim the same. As soon as they smell car air fresheners or motors they get nauseous, before the vehicle even begins to move.

Let me remind you of the orange juice trick over here. If there's nothing you can do about a smell in a car or you're not sure if the car will smell or not, make sure to take along you orange juice so you won't have to sit and smell any of those horrible scents.

20. EXPOSURE THERAPY

Exposure therapy, particularly flooding, should, in my opinion, heal you completely from motion sickness brought on by certain modes of transportation. Why only certain modes and not all modes? That's because whichever movement you expose yourself to that's the kind of movement your body will learn to accept and recognize as something that is part of regular, routine life. If you've been healed from car sickness, it doesn't necessarily mean you've been healed from boat sickness.

A majority of sailors, due to the long times they spend on sea, generally end up adapting so well to the sea, that when they get onto solid ground again they often complain about feeling unsteady. However, even the most seasoned sailors may get seasick when they ride on super rough waters that they are unaccustomed to.

I believe that if you ride in a car long enough you will get healed from car sickness.

However, there is one little catch. If you don't do this part of flooding right, it's likely that you won't be successful in healing yourself.

In psychology, when flooding is used the client may not escape the trigger of his phobia, no matter how high the panic becomes. He needs to just ride out his panic wave, without indulging in a single avoidance behavior or fear relieving activity.

I believe that flooding must work in the same manner in order to heal motion sickness. Once you commit to riding in a vehicle for a certain amount of time, no matter how nauseous you get, you cannot indulge in a single nausea relieving activity. In fact, if you decide to go ahead and subject yourself to flooding, you must temporarily forget all other tricks and techniques on overcoming nausea that I shared with you.

You should not choose a front seat, you should not try to burp away your nausea with a gaseous drink, and you should not try ice packs or hot tea or anything at all to get out of your queasiness. You just ride it out, even if it means vomiting numerous times. (**Take Caution!** Make sure you keep yourself well hydrated with fluids if you vomit often.)

If you're on a boat, you should not run back and forth between the deck and the deep interior belly of the boat, in an attempt to relieve your nausea. If your goal is to be able to ride happily and comfortably on the deck, stay there for the most part of your trip. If you need to go inside for a specific reason, for a game, meal, sleep or to protect yourself from the weather, that's fine. As long as the action is not an attempt to relieve your nausea, it's totally fine to go ahead with it.

I hope you get the idea. No nausea relieving attempts, no matter which mode of transportation you are using. No Dramimine, no ginger flavored candies, no fizzy drinks. Don't have anything with you that you might try to use in a weak moment, to attempt to overcome your nausea.

While I have not tried exposure therapy myself nor can I be sure that it will work for everybody or anybody for that matter, based on the success of exposure therapy in so many different areas of healing, I believe that this has a very big chance of healing motion sickness for good.

CHAPTER 4
MOVIES

While I didn't mention movie induced nausea earlier, I do want to talk about it in this chapter.

The word movie is derived from the word moving picture. Basically any sort of moving picture, in any shape and form, can cause motion sickness.

When I refer to movie sickness I refer to motion sickness brought on by any of the following:

- working on a personal computer
- watching a movie on a small screen
- watching a movie in a standard theater
- watching a movie in an IMAX theater
- playing virtual reality games

Basically any form of watching or interacting with screens can cause horrible motion sickness symptoms.

Can you guess what the cause for this is? At this point, I bet you can.

It's simple. Your body is uncomfortable again.

In travel, your body is stationary and moving at the same time. It's sitting in a seat and at the same time it's sensing motion. When you sit and watch a screen, your body is also stationary and moving at the same time. Well, definitely from your body's perspective. As far as your body is concerned, it's sitting in a seat, and at the same time it's sensing motion. It's getting feedback that it is traveling far distances, through the movement on the screen. So here it is expecting to have a regular everyday visual experience, but instead it's receiving all sorts of funny messages that it is in a place of movement.

What does your body do as a result? It makes you feel sick.

It's interesting. When I first got my computer, I'd become super dizzy whenever I was on it. With time however, that feeling was completely gone. What happened? Natural exposure therapy was at work. I was forced to use my computer, so over time my body just adjusted to that reality. By today my body recognizes computer time as relaxation time!

Now don't think my body is comfortable with *all* screen activity. IMAX theaters are a great trigger for my nausea. It's a great torture chamber for me. This is because my body never adapted to an IMAX theater. Who has an IMAX theater at home? How often does anybody visit an IMAX theater? It is reasonable that most people have adapted to their personal computer screen but will feel sick when watching a movie in an IMAX theater or even in a regular theater. Our bodies are just not used to that sort of viewing!

I believe that Dramimine would work to prevent the histamine your body produces, when you are viewing or interacting with a movie, to have an effect on you. Since Dramimine is not officially made to be used for movie sickness though I suggest you discuss it with a doctor before you decide to take it for movie sickness.

The downside of this is that you cannot take Dramimine long term. So while it might be a good option for that once in a while when you visit an IMAX theater, it's certainly not an option for everyday gaming activities or movie watching.

What should be most effective and can actually heal movie sickness is exposure therapy. It should be way less intense and more comfortable than the therapy you would need to go through to overcome car, air or sea travel. I also believe you can use gradual exposure therapy here as opposed to Flooding. Flooding should definitely bring you successful results, but if you want to be gentler to your senses, you can choose gradual exposure instead.

Here's what you would do:

Let's say you want to become comfortable when playing computer games. No problem. Force yourself to spend one to two straight hours playing on the computer each day for a certain amount of consecutive days.

Once you see that you no longer experience any motion sickness symptoms, you'll know that you're healed. That's it. It's that simple.

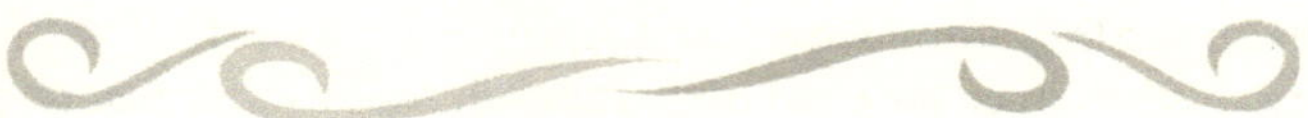

I will leave you now my friend so you can begin implementing some of the tricks and techniques I shared with you here. Let me know how it goes. Reach out to me at indiepenn@gmail.com with all your comments and questions.

Good Luck and Happy Traveling!

www.ingramcontent.com/pod-product-compliance
Lightning Source LLC
Chambersburg PA
CBHW051134250726
48655CB00007B/3049